13.95 6

MW00513475

Also by Anthea Peries

Cancer and Chemotherapy
Coping with Cancer & Chemotherapy Treatment: What You
Need to Know to Get Through Chemo Sessions
Coping with Cancer: How Can You Help Someone with
Cancer, Dealing with Cancer Family Member, Facing Cancer
Alone, Dealing with Terminal Cancer Diagnosis,
Chemotherapy Treatment & Recovery
Chemotherapy Survival Guide: Coping with Cancer &
Chemotherapy Treatment Side Effects

Eating Disorders
Food Cravings: Simple Strategies to Help Deal with Craving
for Sugar & Junk Food
Sugar Cravings: How to Stop Sugar Addiction & Lose Weight
The Immune System, Autoimmune Diseases & Inflammatory
Conditions: Improve Immunity, Eating Disorders & Eating
for Health
Food Addiction: Overcome Sugar Bingeing, Overeating on
Junk Food & Night Eating Syndrome

Food Addiction: Overcoming your Addiction to Sugar, Junk Food, and Binge Eating

Food Addiction: Why You Eat to Fall Asleep and How to Overcome Night Eating Syndrome

Overcome Food Addiction: How to Overcome Food Addiction, Binge Eating and Food Cravings

Healthy Gut: Transform Your Health from the Inside Out, for a Healthy You

Emotional Eating: Stop Emotional Eating & Develop Intuitive Eating Habits to Keep Your Weight Down

Emotional Eating: Overcoming Emotional Eating, Food Addiction and Binge Eating for Good

Food Addiction

Overcoming Food Addiction to Sugar, Junk Food. Stop Binge Eating and Bad Emotional Eating Habits

Food Addiction: Overcoming Emotional Eating, Binge Eating and Night Eating Syndrome

Grief, Bereavement, Death, Loss

Coping with Loss & Dealing with Grief: Surviving Bereavement, Healing & Recovery After the Death of a Loved One

How to Plan a Funeral

Health Fitness

How To Avoid Colds and Flu Everyday Tips to Prevent or Lessen The Impact of Viruses During Winter Season

Quark Cheese
50 More Ways to Use Quark Low-fat Soft Cheese: The Natural Alternative When Cooking Classic Meals

Quark Cheese Recipes: 21 Delicious Breakfast Smoothie Ideas Using Quark Cheese

30 Healthy Ways to Use Quark Low-fat Soft Cheese

Standalone
Family Style Asian Cookbook: Authentic Eurasian Recipes: Traditional Anglo-Burmese & Anglo-Indian

Coping with Loss and Dealing with Grief: The Stages of Grief and 20 Simple Ways on How to Get Through the Bad Days

Table of Contents

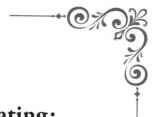

Emotional Eating:

STOP EMOTIONAL EATING & Develop Intuitive Eating Habits to Keep Your Weight Down

Anthea Peries

fashion deemed liable for any hardship or damages that may befall them after undertaking information described herein.

Additionally, the information in the following pages is intended only for informational purposes and should thus be thought of as universal. As befitting its nature, it is presented without assurance regarding its prolonged validity or interim quality. Trademarks that are mentioned are done without written consent and can in no way be considered an endorsement from the trademark holder.

You should seek the medical advice of a professional before embarking on any change to your diet.

Are you an Emotional Eater?

Do you eat anytime you feel upset or happy?

Are you frustrated with yourself, but can't figure out how to fix it?

Does this sound familiar? *You arrive back home from a long day at work. It was stressful, horrible, and all you want to do is curl up on the couch. You know you should eat something healthy for dinner, but you end up eating an entire package of cookies. You feel guilty and shameful after, and the stress is still there. Plus, now you feel physically upset - bloated and fat. Why do you do this to yourself? Why are you like this? How can you change when you don't even know where to start?*

Emotional eating is a thorny issue and one that affects an average of 30% of adults. It can seem very confusing and hard to deal with, and most don't even know they do it!

Emotional Eating: *Stop Emotional Eating & Develop Intuitive Eating Habits to Keep Your Weight Down* can help!

This is a fantastic and comprehensive book, all about how to deal with emotional eating. You can learn so many things that can help you, and things that you'll be able to use both daily and over time. It helps you to develop healthy and lasting habits that get you healthy and in shape.

Within the book are tips, explanations, goals, and counsel including:

- *How to deal with your emotional eating*
- *Tips on dealing with stress*
- *Activities that can replace emotional eating*
- *The Hunger Scale*
- *Healthy foods*
- *Emotional eating triggers*
- *The benefits of journaling*
- *How to lose weight as an emotional eater*
- *Self-care tips*
- *Binge recovery*
- *How to avoid stress*
- *Intuitive eating*
- *Mindful eating*
- *How therapy can help*
- *How social media can help with emotional eating*
- *Meditating*
- *How to treat yourself like royalty*
- *How to connect with other emotional eaters*
- *Your support system*
- *Relaxation techniques*
- *Questions you can ask yourself before eating*

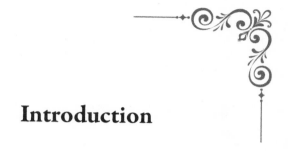

Introduction

CONGRATULATIONS ON downloading *Emotional Eating* and thank you for doing so!

The following chapters will discuss how to stop emotional eating and how to develop intuitive eating habits to keep your weight down.

Emotional Eating can be tough handle. It is emotionally, mentally, and physically taxing, and can last your entire life. Luckily, there are many different tricks and habits you can do that will help out - things that develop over time.

You need to find what works best for you and stick to it. It's hard to develop habits but using the information from this book will help you to succeed.

Just remember that there isn't a quick fix when it comes to emotional eating. It's hard work but work worth doing. This book will help you on the right path towards becoming a healthy eater.

There are plenty of books on the subject on the market, thanks again for choosing this one! Every effort was made to ensure it is full of as much useful information as possible; please enjoy!

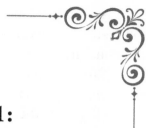

Chapter 1:
Introduction to
Emotional Eating

CUT TO THAT ONE SPECIFIC scene from movies, with the woman crying over a bowl of ice cream and lamenting the terrible thing that just happened. Why does she have the ice cream? Will it solve her problems? Is it going to fix whatever happened to her? Unless she's upset because she wanted a bowl of ice cream, and now has one, then no - ice cream won't actually solve her issue. Then why is she eating it? Sure, ice cream tastes good! It's a big tub of creamy goodness that tastes like a little piece of heaven. But why is she eating it when she's upset? She could do something else to help her feel better, right? She could try activities like calling a friend, writing things down, taking a walk. Doing those things seem like the easy answer but are in actuality pretty tricky.

We are a people of instant gratification, and nothing is more immediate than the good feelings we get from eating something that tastes good. You had a hard day at work? Order pizza for dinner! Is that a bad breakup? Binge out on chips and chocolate! We use food to help with those bad feelings, hoping that they'll go away, even if it's just for a little bit.

Basically, emotional eating is using food to make yourself feel better, even when you're not hungry. It's a way to satisfy emotional needs instead of physical ones, like hunger. And while binge-eating celery might not sound so bad, emotional eaters tend to go straight for the high-carb, high-sugar foods; our bodies crave those types of foods when feeling upset or depressed.

Most people think emotional eating is due to a lack of self-control, but actually, two of the biggest reasons for emotional eating are stress and boredom. It's a sort of automatic reflex; some people don't even realise their eating until after it's happened!

Being stressed out is the more obvious one, but what about boredom? Think about how you sit in front of the TV, binge-watching your favourite show. It's nice having something to munch on while you're just sitting there, right? Or perhaps you can't think of what you want to do. You don't feel like going out; you don't feel like watching TV, you don't really feel like doing anything. But you have this feeling of needing to do something, so you decide to eat. And you're no longer bored, so you just keep eating until past the point of full.

There are many other reasons for emotional eating. You might be feeling depressed, and the food is a type of comfort. Maybe it's a social thing. You're out with your friends, and all of them are ordering dessert, so you have to order dessert. Even though you're feeling overly full, you still order because everyone else did. You could also use emotional eating as a way to celebrate happy news. Food is used as a reward system, so you eat every time you get good news or do something that makes you proud of yourself. It makes for an unhealthy relationship with food. Instead of seeing food as something you need for survival, it's seen as more; something you almost become attached to.

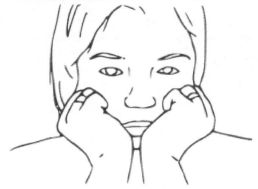

Emotional eating is an addiction, and like any other addiction, it can be challenging to overcome. This book is a way to recognise that you are an emotional eater, and how to deal with overcoming it. There is no 'one right way'. There are many ways and solutions, and hopefully, this book will help you figure out what works best for you.

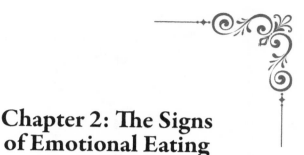

Chapter 2: The Signs of Emotional Eating

SEVERAL SIGNS SHOW you're an emotional eater. Some are in response to positive emotions, and some are in response to negative emotions. And sometimes, it can be difficult to recognise the signs. In fact, you might recognise just one or all of them. As long as you know them in yourself, then you're one step closer to reaching a healthier you!

Eating When Stressed

Probably, the most prominent sign you're an emotional eater is that you eat when stressed. Your stress could come from work, school, or your personal life. Wherever it comes from, your first instinct is to reach for food to deal with all the feelings you're having. While eating, you're able to just focus on the food and forget about what stressed you out in the first place. Basically, you have strong emotions, and the only way you know how to deal with them is by eating. The issue with this is that after you're done eating, the stress is still there. Eating something made you feel better for a while, but now you're feeling overly full and stressed.

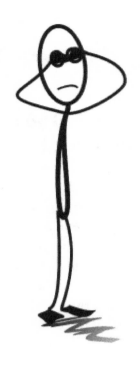

OTHER EMOTIONS

It doesn't have to be stress that affects your eating habits! You could eat when you feel sad, bored, or even happy! Think about all the celebrations you have in your life, and how many include food - birthdays, holidays, also just going out with friends. When at a birthday party, do you feel like you have to eat? It's part of the celebration, so you have to eat in order to properly enjoy yourself, right? What about when you're bored, or even just watching a movie? Let's say you go to the movies with some friends - eating popcorn and candy makes the movie seem so much better. But the movie doesn't change, so wouldn't you still enjoy yourself without the food?

Comfort

You get a particular kind of comfort from eating food, especially ones that have no actual nutritional value. Eating cake feels the same as wrapping yourself up in a comfy blanket or getting a hug. And you don't understand why the food gives you a comforting feeling, but you keep eating because you don't want to lose it. It doesn't even have to be when you're stressed or upset. Maybe it's just a random snowy day, and you want to feel a little comfort and warmth. Instead of drinking hot tea, you decide to eat a piece of pie.

Trouble Losing Weight/Can't Stop Eating

You try to lose weight, but nothing appears to be working. And that upsets you, so you eat comfort food, which makes it even harder to lose weight. And you know what you're eating is terrible for you. It hurts more than helps, but you can't seem to stop yourself because you're so upset. You constantly question yourself about why you can't lose weight, even though deep down you know the answer.

Eat/Think About Food When Full

All you can think about is food, and when your next meal is. You never feel satisfied, even though you definitely ate enough during your last meal to be full. You could be out and about running errands, doing completely normal daily tasks. At this juncture, all you can really think about is eating that piece of cake you have at home. You could be at a restaurant with friends, and decide to get another entrée, not for right now, but for dinner later. And you can't stop thinking about it once you get home, so, instead of waiting for dinner, you decide to go ahead and eat it, even though you literally just had lunch.

Social

You eat a lot in social settings, mainly because others are eating and not because you're actually hungry. A typical example is while attending a festival or state fair. They always have booths and tents with tons of food. People are all around, eating amazing-looking things. These include home-made pie, turkey legs, home-made ice cream, soft pretzels, etc. And we tell ourselves that part of going to fairs and festivals is to eat the food. It's the social norm and not eating the various treats will make you stand out in a negative way. Trying a little bit of the different things is fine. However, the problem starts when you end up eating plateful after plateful because everyone else is. This is just because it's the 'thing to do'.

Chapter 3: The Dangers of Emotional Eating

WHEN FIRST LOOKING at it, emotional eating might not seem that bad. A piece of chocolate after something upsets you can actually be good, right? Research has even shown that one piece of chocolate can be healthy for you! So that means it's ok to eat it, right? Also, you were feeling upset, and now feel so much better. You can focus on the rest of your day in a positive light, and things are great! So why is it thought to be such a bad thing?

The first thing to ask yourself is why you were so upset in the first place? Eating that piece of chocolate made you feel way better, but did it solve the reason that made you are upset? What if whatever happened to upset you occurs again? And it repeats itself again, and again? If all you do to solve it is eating a piece of chocolate, it'll never be addressed. Also, you'll end up stuck in a continuous loop of upset feelings being covered up by emotional eating.

This leads you to be emotionally dependent on food. Anytime something bad happens, you use food to cover up those negative feelings, and just keep continuing the self-destructive loop. Food becomes your crutch and develops into unhealthy eating habits.

Doing these things and feeling this way creates the illusion of happiness. Emotional eating never actually solves anything, covers it up. Whatever happiness you're feeling is temporary and false. And worst of all, whatever made you feel so upset is still out there and still exists.

Which means it can, and will, come back into your life whether you like it or not. And what's worse in that these emotions will come back even stronger than before. You were stressed, so you ate something unhealthily. Now you're feeling stress, and guilty, ashamed, embarrassed, etc. You feel so much worse than before, and nothing got solved. Dealing with the issue head-on instead of covering it up with induced happiness is much better for your mental and emotional health.

Your physical health is also at risk. The most obvious is, of course, weight gain. This puts you at risk for diabetes, heart attacks, and numerous other health issues. In a way, you're abusing your own body. The types of foods emotional eaters typically go for are high in carbs and sugars. In addition to being the normally bad practice for you, foods like that also create fatigue and depression.

Think of your body like a car. If you put the wrong gas in it and drive it around without taking care of it, your car won't run or will even break down when you least expect it. Your body is the same way. Emotional eating puts unnecessary wear and tear on our bodies, forcing them to break down faster than we would like.

Emotional eating can also cause something called Mindless Eating. This phenomenon happens when we make food choices but aren't really aware of it. Basically, we don't think about what we're eating; we just eat it. When a person eats because of emotions, they don't really think about what they're doing. They choose foods that are unhealthy and end up eating a lot more calories. When someone eats because of normal hunger pains, they think about what they want to eat and make better choices.

There's also the implication of your children's eating behaviours. You might think that your eating habits only affect you, but it's just not true for those with children. Children mimic eating habits from a very young age. They also pick up behaviours, patterns, and food choices from their parents. Think of it as the phrase "learning by example".

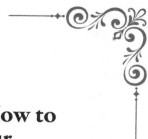

Chapter 4: How to Find Your Emotional Eating Triggers

A TRIGGER IS A FEELING or situation, which directly causes you to eat emotionally. Different persons have different triggers that affect their overeating habit. Recognizing these triggers can help you avoid or solve them before the feeling of wanting to eat happens.

So how do we recognize our triggers? The first thing to do is look at what you feel when you emotionally eat. Are you eating because you're bored? When stressed? When happy? If emotional eating makes you happy, what were you feeling before you started eating? By looking at the feelings you were having previously, you can narrow down what exact feeling you were having that caused you to overeat.

Looking at the cause of the feeling is helpful to understand why you're an emotional eater. Do you only overeat after talking with a specific friend? Is it after you go through your bills? Or after coming home from a hard day at work?

Technology is also a popular trigger for emotional eaters. We just sit around, watching television, or videos on our phones. Our minds are focused on what we're watching, but our bodies are just sitting still. We're used to having more physical stimulation, such as walking or typing at the computer, so sitting still like that is actually pretty difficult, and we compensate for that by eating.

Here are a few triggers listed out, see if you recognize any of them within yourself:

Stress or boredom

Eating can be a way to relieve stress and boredom. Maybe you feel unfulfilled or unsatisfied with your life. Maybe you're constantly stressed from work, and you think the only way to deal with it is by eating. When emotionally eating, you feel as if you can stuff those feelings down so far that you don't have to deal with them.

Socially

Getting together with friends can be a lot of fun. You're out for a good time, and you just want to let loose. Maybe everyone decides to order a ton of food, and you feel like you have to keep up. Or everyone is ordering dessert, so you feel the pressure to order dessert too. It's very easy to give in when you are with a group of friends.

A good example is that your friend wants to order something but wants to share it. You weren't planning on getting anything else, but she insists that you share it with her. You give in because she's your friend and you don't want to feel left out. Later, you're stuck eating something you really didn't want or need.

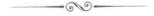

CHILDHOOD HABITS

It's entirely possible and likely that your emotional eating issues came from childhood habits. Think back to your childhood, and how food was presented to you. Did your parents use it as a reward? Did you get ice cream every time you got an A? Maybe they used treats to cheer you up when you were sad. It's also possible that your eating habits are fueled by nostalgia. You have all these fond memories of family dinners or baking and eating cookies, and you try to recapture that love by overeating now.

Being too hungry

Do you try to eat healthy for breakfast and lunch, only to completely binge once dinner rolls around? Maybe you think skipping breakfast is the best option because it's "healthier". You go about your day, getting hungrier and hungrier and thinking you'll be fine. You feel that you can control your hunger. But once you get home, you realize that you're starving, and eat so much that you're feeling way too full after. The best thing to do is not skip meals and have small snacks throughout the day. If you actually feed your body at normal intervals, you'll get home in the evening and feel a little hungry. However, this is not enough to binge.

Eating in the evening

Evening and late night can be a big trigger. Most people think of it as their "me time", or a time to "treat myself". The reason is that it's the only time they get to themselves all day. With that kind of thinking, it's incredibly easy to overindulge in food. Eating in the evening also happens because of being too tired. You might be very tired but don't want to go to bed. So, note that eating something will help to keep you awake.

Work treats

It's always there. That box of donuts your co-worker brings in every day. It's so tempting, and you know it's bad for you. But work is always so busy, and you get really hungry throughout the day, so eating what's there in the office is just convenient. It's so easy to just grab at what's there until you realize it's the end of the day and you've eaten three donuts. This can often be a tough one to deal with. You should keep in mind that you're probably not the only one at the office who's trying to deal with staying away from those unhealthy treats.

Too much going on. Perhaps there is just so much going on in your life at the moment. You're trying to juggle five different things, and it's getting to be almost impossible to keep up with everything. Eating helps slow it all down, just a little, and makes everything seem better. It's an easy way to find comfort or even a much-needed energy boost. And while the immediate effects are subtle, the long-term ones aren't worth all the negative consequences that come later. Learning how to deal with your busy schedule and figuring out how to cut things back will assist you to take back control of your life once more.

Chapter 5: How to Stop Emotional Eating

IT CAN BE CHALLENGING to stop emotional eating. Overeating has become a crutch, something that makes you feel good about yourself. And, at least for a short time, it takes away the stress and pain that you're trying to deal with. That being said, being an emotional eater is not healthy, and finding a way to stop it is the best option for a healthier life.

The first thing you need to do is figure out your emotional eating triggers. They say knowledge is power, and while knowing what the trigger is won't stop your emotional eating, it's the first step to becoming a healthier you. Your triggers could be just one thing or a number of things. If you're not sure of what they are, try writing down anytime you feel hungry, and what happened immediately before. Maybe you were just talking to a friend on the phone, and they caused you to feel stressed. Perhaps you're watching TV and need the act of moving your hands around, and the only thing you can think of to help is eating.

Once you figure out your triggers, the next step is to understand the why of them. I spoke a little about this in the previous chapter. Looking at the cause of the feeling you get helps you to understand why you're an emotional eater.

For example, let's say you're at a work birthday party. And there's a big, tasty looking birthday cake for everyone to share. Of course, you think that it's only polite to eat a piece or two, even if you're not hungry. But some people aren't eating cake, and when asked why, they say it's because they're not hungry. So why do you feel like you have to eat that cake? Is it just because it was there? Or it is because you can only celebrate and be happy when eating food?

The next big step to stop emotional eating is to separate eating from your triggers. I know, I know, easier said than done! But you've done the hardest step already. That is figuring out your triggers and where they come from. Let's use the birthday cake example again. It's a celebration, and that means celebrating with food, right? Instead of using food to celebrate, relish in the happiness and good news. You can do that either with friends or on your own. Whichever you choose that allows you to embrace the joy at a deeper level, one that lasts much longer than that piece of cake.

Sometimes we have to address the triggers themselves instead of detaching. A significant example of this is stress management. You can't merely detach from stress; it's always going to be there. In fact, it would be extremely unhealthy to just disconnect from your feelings! While stress is a negative emotion, it's a good thing that you feel it. What you can do is to choose a healthier way to deal with it instead of eating. Understand that stress is just another emotion, and there are ways to deal with feelings. You need to find what works best for you - exercise, journaling, talking with someone, even deep breathing and meditation.

You might have more than one trigger, which means it could take a while before you're entirely rid of emotional eating. And that's ok! Just focus on each step for each trigger, and you'll get there.

Chapter 6: Choosing Healthier Foods as an Emotional Eater

IT CAN BE TOUGH TO quit cold turkey when you're an emotional eater. You keep getting craving after craving and doing nothing seems to add more stress. Then you end up binge eating super unhealthy foods, and it becomes an endless loop.

One great way to resolve that issue is by replacing junk food with healthy options! This, in itself, can also be very difficult. Who wants celery sticks when you can have yummy chocolate?

The key is to fill up with protein, which helps get rid of those pesky carbohydrate cravings. One great snack for that is Ants on a Log. I know, I just mentioned how celery isn't tasty. But you should fill it with peanut butter and raisins, and you've got a fantastic snack that's not just for kids!

Another fantastic snack is making your own DIY snack bites. You can just throw them in your mouth like a handful of popcorn, and they fill you up in a much healthier way. Just mix dates, nuts, and nut butter to create a healthy, TV binging, worthy snack.

What about satisfying your sweet tooth? Honey is a great healthy alternative to processed sugars and can be used in a variety of ways. One great one is making peanut butter and banana toast. Just sprinkle some honey on it for that extra sweetness!

Now, here's some really good news - you don't have to give up chocolate completely! So exciting! Dark chocolate is good for you and has been shown to reduce stress levels. Dark chocolate almond is a great snack, and when portioned correctly, can make for a tasty treat.

Let's say you're binge-watching your favourite show and are really craving some snacks. Veggies and dip is a great healthy snack that provides impressive nutrients without the unhealthy problems that come with other snack foods. Hummus makes for a fantastic dip and goes great with carrots, celery, and bell peppers.

Are you in the mood for snack food but not boring veggies? Try Curry Roasted Chickpeas! It makes a great alternative to chips and is super easy to make! Just cook in a saucepan and add your favourite spices!

You could also have a fruit parfait instead of ice cream, trail mix for a tasty snack, and even tea and flavoured water! Sometimes our bodies seem hungry, but it's actually mistaken for dehydration. It's extremely important to drink plenty of water, and an excellent substitute for sodas is flavored seltzer water. It hydrates and fills you up, which helps with cravings.

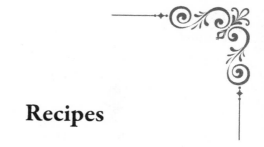

Recipes

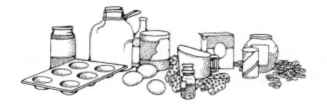

ANTS ON A LOG:

Ingredients:

Celery

Peanut Butter (or alternative)

Raisins

Directions:

Cut celery into bite-sized pieces

Put peanut butter into celery gap

Place raisins on peanut butter

Enjoy!

DIY Snack Bites:

Ingredients:

1/2 cup chopped dates

1/4 cup rolled oats

1/2 cup nut butter

Directions:

Mix together

Roll into bite-sized balls

Enjoy!

Peanut Butter and Banana Toast:

Ingredients:

1 slice whole wheat bread

1 tbs peanut butter

1/2 banana

Drizzle of honey

Directions:

Toast bread

Spread peanut butter on toast

Slice banana and place on top of the peanut butter

Sprinkle with honey

Enjoy!

Curry Roasted Chickpeas:

Ingredients:

Olive Oil

Eden Organic No Salt Added Chickpeas

Curry Powder

Cumin

Paprika

Garlic Powder

Sea Salt

Directions:

Heat 1 and 1/2 tsp olive oil in a saucepan over medium-high heat

Add 1/2 cup rinsed, drained, and dried chickpeas

Cook 5 to 7 minutes, turning frequently

Toss with 1/2 tsp curry powder, a generous pinch of cumin, garlic powder, paprika, and sea salt

Enjoy!

Here are a few more snacks that are healthy and are great replacements for unhealthy ones! Some of these snacks actually require you to use your hands, like pistachios and oranges. That helps when you're the type of emotional eater who tends to eat because they're bored and wants something to do with their hands:

- *Popcorn*
- *Pistachios*
- *Blueberries*
- *Edamame*
- *Orange*
- *Kale Chips*
- *Walnuts*
- *Herbal Teas*

Chapter 7: Common Emotional Eating Triggers to Avoid

ONE OF THE MOST SHARED emotional eating triggers is **boredom**. People tend to live very stimulating lives; we go to work and interact with our coworkers, we take vacations, we go on daily trips (like the grocery store), even surfing the web on our phones can be very stimulating. We're constantly surrounded by things thrown in our faces, by things going on around us. So when we have a few moments just to sit down and take a breather, sometimes we don't really know what to do with ourselves. We feel as if we have to be doing something, and use eating as a way to fill the void. If there's nothing else to do, we might as well eat something! It not only relieves our boredom but also makes us feel better too.

Habit is another common trigger. Think about this. When you get home from work, it's usually about dinner time, so you make and eat dinner. Doing this becomes a habit, one that makes sense. But it becomes such a habit, which you start eating every time you get home from somewhere, no matter the time. Coming back from the grocery store at 2 pm? Your mind and body are in the habit of making food when you get home, so you decide to eat something. Except it's not a regular meal time, so you make a snack, one that might not be very healthy. Or even to make a complete meal, which your body doesn't need at that time. And it's tough to break a habit, so it just seems easier to go with it.

What about **fatigue**? It's so easy to overeat when you're feeling down and tired. Let's say you have the day off and don't feel like doing anything. This is completely fine. It's your day off, and you deserve some downtime! You decide to spend the whole day binge-watching your favourite show. After some time, you start feeling tired, even though you've just been lying on the couch all day. You don't feel like actually doing anything, so figure out the best way to pep yourself up is by eating. Even though you're not hungry and don't need food at the moment, you still end up eating a whole bag of chips.

Another example is getting tired at work. You're on your break and start feeling tired around 3. You still have a few hours left but need a pick-me-up. And instead of drinking tea or even just water, which would definitely help, you decide to eat something. And you have a little energy, but it doesn't last very long, and now you're feeling tired and overly full.

One of the hardest common emotional eating triggers is **social influences**. It's fun to go out with friends, but it's very easy to overeat when doing so. You meet early for drinks and eat a little something at the bar. Then decide to go to a restaurant for dinner. And then decide to go out to another place, where they might have amazing nachos. From there to another location, and another place, and another, until you've realized that you've eaten something at every single place.

Or maybe you're meeting with a group kind of late and decide to eat dinner at home to save money. But then you get there, and everyone is eating, so you feel like you have to order something too. And now you've spent the money, so you feel like you have to eat it; otherwise, it's money wasted. And then everyone orders dessert, and you feel as if everyone will think it odd if you don't eat any. But now you've eaten two dinners and dessert, which is something your body doesn't need. This one is the most difficult because it involves your friends and wanting to fit in.

A great way to avoid this is by having one of your friends being your accountability partner. Someone you know will be within the group and can back you up when you're thinking about joining everyone else for dinner even though you don't need it.

Then there's the feeling of **comfort** that food can give you. It's so easy to use food as a comfort, especially if it's something you grew up around. Maybe your parents used food as a reward system or soothing technique. Would you get ice cream if you had a bad day at school? Or what about the trope of eating ice cream when your significant other has broken up with you. Even the weather can affect how food comforts us! Who doesn't love a mug of hot chocolate when it's snowing outside? Or a colossal snow cone when it's a simmering summer day?

The main issue is that we start to rely on food to give us comfort that we can't find elsewhere. And we feel comforted for a while, but whatever was bothering us before will definitely come back because food can only do so much. Eating can't actually get rid of our problems.

Stress is a big emotional eating trigger, if not the biggest one. Maybe you just had an argument with your best friend. Maybe you're dealing with financial issues. Maybe you're worried about your job. We've all been there! You don't like dealing with the negative emotions, and eating has a sort of soothing quality to it. So instead of dealing with your stress, you start binging. And for a while, things seem ok. You're focused on the food, and things don't seem that bad. But once you're done eating, all the stress and unpleasant feelings have come back.

The best thing to do is find something else besides food to help with your stress, something that's much healthier than emotional eating. Finding something to replace stress can really help in the long run.

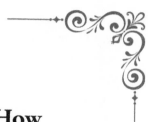

Chapter 8: How Journaling Can Help You with Emotional Eating

ONE FANTASTIC COPING strategy for emotional eating is journaling. Writing things down can help you to understand a situation. Using it for emotional eating can pinpoint instances when you get the sudden urge to eat. You can figure out whether you're hungry because of actual hunger pains or a specific emotional situation.

You can also use journaling to track behaviour patterns, such as hunger levels. On a scale from 1 to 10, how hungry are you? If it's just 1 or 2, then do you really need to eat, or is it just habit to eat every little time you feel hungry? Start writing down your level on the hunger scale every time you feel hungry. You'll start to notice patterns and be able to tell around what time every day you're actually hungry. Using that information, you can preemptively eat something healthy so you won't over eat every time you decide to skip a meal.

You can also track what you're doing at the moment you start feeling hungry. Maybe you are sitting in a work meeting and realise that you always begin to munch on a snack because you're sitting there bored. Or you can track what you are precisely feeling at the moment. You can begin to realise that you only overeat when you are happy, sad, bored etc., and compensate for that by emotional eating.

A creative use for journaling is brainstorming ideas. You can think up ways to replace eating, once you figure out what you are feeling at that exact moment. Let's use boredom as an example. You're sitting there, watching a TV show. And while you are not exactly bored, you still feel like you need to do something with your hands. So, of course, your mind immediately jumps to food. You pick out a yummy snack and just start binging. Or maybe you're not watching TV, but just sitting there and eating because you can't think of anything else to do. Using your journal, you can think up different and creative ways to replace the binge eating. Maybe try knitting, colour in a colouring book, or reading a new book. If you need something to do with your hands while watching a TV show or a movie, try twirling a pen or playing with a fidget spinner. There are a lot of different gadgets and things you can try out instead of eating.

Basically, just write down a ton of different things you can try, even ones that you think you wouldn't like. And start doing them every time you start feeling stressed or bored. Keep working out things from your list, and soon enough you'll have a new hobby and will start getting healthier. And depending on what you decide, like going on a walk, you could even start losing weight!

Even just writing things down can help! Instead of eating, pick up a pen and start writing. It doesn't also have to make sense; just start writing what you did that day or even a list of all the words you know. If you hate writing, you can always try drawing. It does not have to be super amazing; just little doodles will work. This is as long as you try redirecting your emotions into something healthier than binge eating. Bottling up stress and strong feelings isn't healthy and writing everything down is a positive way to let your emotions out.

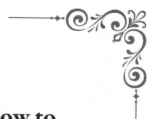

Chapter 9: How to Lose Weight When You Are an Emotional Eater

LOSING WEIGHT AS AN emotional eater is probably one of the hardest things to cope with. You try to lose weight, but it's not working, so you're stressed. And when you're stressed, you eat. It's a vicious cycle and an unending loop. How are you supposed to lose weight?

Working out is the obvious choice, of course. But there are also different ways that can help you to stop overeating, which will, in turn, help you to lose weight.

Again, we take into account your triggers. Take a minute and think about why you're suddenly craving something. Are you upset? Are you stressed? Are you bored? Instead of eating, try journaling. As said in the previous chapter, journaling is a fantastic way to cope with emotional eating. It's a way to process your stress and emotions in a healthy manner. Accepting your emotions also helps. Accept that you're upset, frustrated, or angry, instead of trying to cover it up with food. Take a long deep breath and say "I am angry" as you let it out. Even, you need to state why you are feeling this way. You can end up having an entire discussion with yourself! It might seem a little silly, but if it works then why not do it? It's a good way to help you accept your emotions and let them go without holding on to them.

Another good to help you lose weight is to think about what you're eating. And that doesn't mean focus on diets/fads, but concentrate specifically on your food. Instead of eating as much as you can, think about what you're putting in your mouth.

Try these different tricks the next time you are eating:

Counting bites. Focus on each bite as you're chewing. Count how many bites it takes for this specific mouthful. Do the same thing with the next mouthful and see if it takes the same number of bites or if it's different. Counting bites force you to pause a little while eating, which in turn help you not to overeat.

Put your fork down in between bites. Instead of holding your fork in your hand the whole time, try putting it down while you're chewing. Put the food in your mouth, place the fork on your plate or napkin, and focus on counting your bites. Once you've swallowed, pick your fork back up, and repeat the process.

Try to figure out all the different ingredients in your food. Does your food taste salty? Is it spicy or sweet? Maybe there's a specific spice, but you can't quite figure it out. Try focusing on it with each bite and see if you can pinpoint which spice it is. Don't just focus on the ingredients either; is your food chewy or crunchy? Is it totally soft, or are there hard bits in it? By focusing on this specifically on your food, you eat a little more slowly, which in turn will help you to feel fuller in a faster amount of time.

Take smaller bites. Sometimes we're so hungry that we just scarf down our food in these huge bites, and don't even notice how full we are until we're completely done. And most of the time, we end up feeling overly full and lament on why we ate so much. Instead, try cutting your bites in half. Put the normal amount you usually do on your fork or spoon, but then put half of it back on your plate. Do this with every bite, and you'll realise that you feel full a lot sooner than you normally would. You'll probably even have leftovers on your plate!

Research has shown that eating slower helps you feel full faster, which means those who eat slowly don't overeat. So really concentrate on your food. Don't split your focus with other things, like TV. Try sitting down at a table and focus only on your food. If you're focusing on something else while you eat, it's extremely easy just to keep putting food in your mouth without realising that you're overeating.

You could also take a break before eating. It's possible your body is using hunger pains as a way to tell you something else.

When you start feeling hungry, try these things first -

Take 5 minutes off and do something else. It doesn't have to be anything special! You could start a load of laundry, wash dishes, go on social media, even watch a YouTube video. The most important thing is to take those 5 minutes for something else. It's entirely possible that after those 5 minutes are up, you won't actually feel hungry anymore. This is especially good for those who are emotional eaters due to boredom.

Take a step back and analyze your emotions. As an emotional eater, it's more likely that you're feeling hungry due to some overwhelming emotions. Before getting something to eat, focus on what you're feeling. Are you stressed, upset, maybe even happy? There are other ways to help you get through these feelings besides eating. Try one of the many different solutions first, like journaling or meditating.

Drink water. Maybe all you need is a glass of water! It's actually very easy to mistake dehydration for hunger, so drink your water first. It will help you decide if you're truly hungry or not. It's important to get enough water, and most people don't actually drink the right amount. So try drinking 8 ounces of water first and see if you are still hungry.

Try exercising or an activity. One of the most significant ways to lose weight for emotional eaters is replacing eating with some sort of exercise or activity. It doesn't have to be jogging or joining a gym unless you like those types of thing. Honestly, it really depends on what you're looking for. If you're bored, then something a little faster paced would make sense; exercise, watch funny videos, play with your pet/kids, dance to music, etc.

This could be something with high stimulation that helps you to forget your cravings. But if you're stressed, then utilizing something relaxing would be extremely beneficial. Massaging yourself or getting a professional one, taking a bath, aromatherapy, listening to music, and soaking in a hot tub are all great relaxation examples.

Some of these examples might seem counter-productive. You're probably asking yourself how it's even possible to lose weight by giving yourself a massage! However, all these are a way to redirect your strong feelings of hunger. Trying one of these is a healthy way to cope with your emotions and will stop you from emotionally eating. This will, in turn, help you to lose weight!

Chapter 10: Tips to Reduce Daily Stress

STRESS IS EVERYWHERE and something we experience every day. These include stress at work, sitting in traffic, dealing with financial issues, and working out relationship problems. It just keeps adding up more and more all day long, until you're ready to explode by the end of the day. And how is this stress dealt with? Is it by overeating, which just adds to the stress in the long-term?

Trying to find something to help with your stress can be stressful in itself. It's hard to know where even to start, and how to keep up with it. And an added bonus is trying to find something that works specifically for you. One person might be able to go jogging to help deal with their stress, but maybe that option doesn't work for you.

Here's a list of tips and tricks for dealing with your daily stress:

Hang Out With Friends

Hanging out with friends is a great way to help with your stress. They help make you feel better and get you laughing, which helps immensely with stress. Meeting up with a friend for lunch can help you to take a break from a stressful workday. You end up having a good time and go back to the office a lot happier. The feeling is almost like you took a nice nap; you just feel so well rested and ready to accomplish anything!

Going out with friends for the evening is a great way to unwind and talk about how hard your day was. Friends make great sounding boards, and you'll be able to talk about your pushy boss all you want. You're able to get all your stress out by talking, which means it won't happen by eating. And you don't have to spend a ton of money to go out and have fun!

You and your friends can find something free around town, like a local festival. Most cities have art events or farmer's markets that are usually free to enter. And there's an added bonus going to a farmer's market - you can pick up some fantastically healthy food! If you're more of a homebody, you can invite a few friends over instead. You and your friends can watch a movie together or have a fun game night.

Or even try something new! Instead of just watching a movie with your friends, maybe have a painting night. Similar to those painting party places, you and your friends can set up canvases and paint together. Not only are you reducing your stress by having fun with your friends, but you're also getting your emotions out through painting!

Something to remember when considering this trick is that studies show being with people we care about releases hormones which allow us to feel good. So scientifically speaking, it's actually healthier for you to be with friends. Many of those who are depressed tend to be alone. It's difficult for them to be around people but doing so can have a strong positive impact on them. Something as simple as hugging a loved one can help you feel so much better and less stressed and help you to restrain from emotionally eating.

Meditate/Take A Break

Meditating isn't just for Yogis and hippies anymore! It can be an incredibly healthy way to reflect on and center your emotions. Take some time alone to center your thoughts. Get into a comfortable position, whether sitting or lying down on your bed and just reflect. You can count your breaths or the cracks on the ceiling; as long as you're taking time away from your busy schedule just to breathe.

Re-centering your mind and thoughts can really help you to feel lighter and not as stressed. It also can help you to figure out an answer to a problem that you've been dealing with. Sometimes when we focus on one thing, the back of our minds are working out the answer to a problem. So focusing on meditation allows your mind to take a break and you could come out of it with the answer you needed!

Get Moving

You don't have to run 10 miles to feel the benefit of physical activity. And the last thing you probably feel like doing when stressed is getting up and moving around. But physical activity releases endorphins, which makes you feel great! And luckily, it doesn't have to be anything strenuous or difficult.

Some great examples of daily things you can use to be a little more physical than normal are:

Parking in a spot that's further from the store: This forces you to walk just a little bit further than normal. It's really not that bad and think about what those little extra steps can do! Our minds tend to focus better when we take a few minutes break from our busy schedules. Those few extra steps are a great way to relax for a minute, and just focus on what's going on around us. Look at the cars you're walking past, look at the clouds in the sky, or even count your steps. It's almost like a way to "restart" your mental state and helps you not to be as stressed. But what happens if it's raining? Maybe try challenging yourself! Is it really so bad to walk a little in the rain? You can always use an umbrella, and rain is just water. Getting a little wet isn't the end of the world and might feel very refreshing!

Try using the stairs. If your destination is on floor 2 or 3, why not just use the stairs? If you're not sure if you can make it or not, then try going down the stairs at first. Descending on stairs is always easier than going up. It's a great way to get in better shape, and a good way to get you used to take the stairs instead of the elevator or escalator. In all honesty, it will probably be difficult at first. If you're used to the elevator, stairs can be a challenge. But once you're used to it, you feel so much better, and it's a fantastic little exercise you can do almost every day. If you find it especially challenging, try counting the steps. How many does it take to get to your floor? Counting will make it seem like it's going a little faster. It also helps you focus on something other than how much your legs hurt.

If you're the type that hates all form of exercise, try something a little different - dancing to music! It's something you can do anytime and anywhere. If you're especially bold, you can dance-walking down the street while listening to music on your headphones. If you're like most people though, dancing in your living room makes a great alternative. You can put on your favorite tunes, and just start moving around. It doesn't have to look nice, and you definitely don't have to dance like a professional ballerina. Even if it's just swaying back and forth, it'll get you moving and focused on something other than your stress. You can even look into dance classes at your local community center. It brings the social aspect into it, which can also help with stress. Usually, you can find a lot of different types of classes. If you think you'll just be terrible at the more structured ones, like tap or jazz, try a free movement class. It's literally just a bunch of people dancing however they want to music. So basically what you'd be doing in your living room, but with other people!

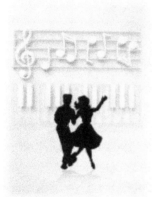

All of these things could take just a few minutes out of your day. They don't require a lot of work, time, or money, but will leave you feeling so much better.

Volunteering

This one might seem silly at first - how can volunteering make me feel less stressed? But actually, it can have a really good impact on how you feel!

You experience social interactions with the other volunteers, which helps you to feel connected with others. You feel a certain 'togetherness' when volunteering with others as if you're all connected in a very special way. It's a great way to make new friends and being in a group setting tends to help you forget about the reason you're so stressed.

There's most likely a physical aspect involved. You could be serving food to the homeless, so you're continually lifting a spoon or ladle. It doesn't seem like much but lifting a heavy spoon over and over again can be a pretty good workout for your arms! You might have to move boxes around or sort through piles of clothes. And of course, depending on who you're volunteering for, you might have to actually build houses and fix household maintenance issues.

All of these things get you up and moving around, which is good for you physically. It's also a great way to take your mind off your own emotional issues. Moving around helps you focus on something other than your stress, and after you're done, you leave feeling amazing because you helped others. And sometimes we take a look at how others live and realize that our problems might not seem so bad. Even if it's just once a month, volunteering can be very beneficial, and a great way to put things into perspective.

Hobbies

Think about something you've always wanted to try. Maybe learning how to knit, learning a new language, or building model planes. Maybe even learning how to put those little sailboats in those even smaller glass bottles! Think about all the things out there that you don't know how to do. It actually adds up to a lot; most people know a lot about a very small amount of subjects. There are plenty of things out there that you can try. Think about how accomplished you'll feel after learning a new language! And what doors learning a new hobby will open. Leaning a new language makes it easier to travel. You're able to learn the culture of a new country and speak with the locals. Plus, everyone is very impressed when someone can speak a different language. Or you can take classes on how to knit and meet new friends. Maybe you even find something you enjoy doing so much that you're able to turn it from a hobby to a business! Your life flips complete upside down; now you're no longer dreading going into work, but actually enjoying it! Your life is no longer stressful, so you don't really emotionally eat, which in turn makes you so much healthier. All because you decided to try a new hobby!

Doing something you love will help you feel so better and help reduce your daily stress. Let's say you come home from a horrible day at work. You're tired, hungry, and all you feel like doing is curling up on the couch and binge eating that bag of chips. Instead, take 15 minutes to work on a hobby. It doesn't have to be a long time, just a simple 15 minutes. Try curling up on the couch in your pyjamas with your knitting supplies! After those 15 minutes, you'll feel a little more centered. You de-stressed in a healthy way and feel so much better emotionally. Because of this, you're able to focus on getting a real meal for dinner started.

Fun!

Don't forget about having fun! It's very easy to get caught up in our busy lives, which makes us forget to just focus on what's going on around us. Start looking up different events going on in your city. You don't have to spend a lot of money; most cities have free festivals and farmer's markets. You can try going to an open mic comedy night. Depending on the season, most parks have outdoor movie nights or a concert series; you can bring your blanket and lay out on the grass. If you're more of an introvert, try something that's fun you can do at home. The important thing is to take time for yourself, no matter how selfish you might think you're being. You are the best you when you're doing well emotionally, and the only way to get there is by taking care of yourself. Every day, you should take some time to relax, to do something you enjoy, and to laugh. It might seem cliché? but laughing actually helps to reduce stress, so it's important to laugh every single day! Maybe it's watching your favourite YouTube videos; maybe it's reading your favourite comic book. You can even buy a few kid toys and try them out. Driving a remote-controlled car around your house can be a lot of fun, especially when you have pets! In fact, playing with your pets can be very fun, and is a great way to help reduce stress.

Chapter 11: Why You Should Journal If You Are an Emotional Eater

IN CHAPTER 8, YOU READ how journaling can help with emotional eating. In this chapter, we'll discuss in more detail exactly why you should journal. How important it is, and what exactly happens when you do it.

Journaling might seem silly; after all, isn't it something only teenage girls do? If you want to write down the name of your crush surrounded by a heart, then, by all means, do so! However, since you are trying to focus on the emotional eating aspect of things, definitely consider writing more than that.

Journaling in itself is very beneficial; writing down your thoughts can be very cathartic and a great way to center yourself. It's also good for accountability; by writing down what you've eaten for the day, you can see exactly how much is due to emotional eating. Sometimes it's hard to keep track of what you eat all day; you get caught up in your life and don't realise what you're munching on throughout the day. Sometimes people need things to be written down to help them understand. So by writing it down, you can see how it all adds up. It becomes exact and sort of 'set in stone', instead of the more abstract form of just thinking about it.

Emotional eaters are prone to stress, depression, and numerous other emotions. Compared with eating, journaling is the better of solutions for dealing with all of these intrusive emotions. This might sound a little sappy, but a journal is like having a friend that listens to every single thought you have, without any judgment or backtalk. You're free to say exactly what you want, how you want it. Need to complain about your boss? Want to talk about how your family is always super passive-aggressive and won't leave you alone about your life choices? Then write it down! You're the only one who sees what you've written, so why wouldn't you take advantage of that!

What if you're not a great writer? You definitely don't have to be Shakespeare, but what if you just completely and totally hate writing? If that's an issue, then there are other things you can try. Drawing is a great alternative, and again, you don't have to be a pro! You can just doodle out your feelings. Think about it like this - you're extremely stressed and can't think of anything but your stress. You open your journal, but you can't think of anything to write. That's how stressed you are! So just take the pencil/pen and start making lines. They don't have to be anything spectacular or even specific, just squiggles on a page. The more you do it; the more your stress is disappearing. Even something as simple as doodling can help to relieve strong negative emotions!

Journaling is also useful to keep ideas in. Eating healthy in general is a good idea, and not just for emotional eaters. But it can be difficult to keep track of recipes and meal ideas. Why not use your journal for that? You can start writing down your favourite recipes, and what works and what doesn't. Maybe you tried to make something but can't stand a specific spice it uses. Instead of never trying it again, make changes to the recipe and record those changes in your journal! Again, it also brings in that accountability aspect. If you write down a recepe, you're more likely to use it. If you write down specific goals, you're more likely to do them. Writing things down cements them and helps them to stay in your mind easier. You're less likely to forget something that you've written down.

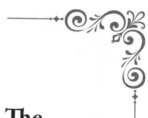

Chapter 12: The Difference between Hunger and Emotional Hunger

YOU CAN THINK OF THIS as very literal - hunger references when your stomach is growling for a true need of food and having actual hunger pains, and emotional hunger refers to when you eat in response to a feeling.

Real hunger is something that doesn't necessarily have to be fixed right away. You can often skip a meal or two without any major side effects; you might be a little faint or fatigued, but still doing all right. You eat just as much as your stomach can take and are able to stop eating once you feel full. Most people's stomachs are the size of their fist, so you're able to eat a well-proportioned meal, and not feel hungry afterwards. Also, you feel the need to eat, but not one specific food. You might be craving a certain thing for dinner, but if you don't get it, then it's not that big of a deal. Whatever food you have will actually satisfy you, and you don't get that feeling of guilt after eating.

Emotional hunger is something that happens because of a strong feeling, which can be either positive or negative. You eat when you're feeling stressed, and you eat when you're feeling happy. It also involves craving a specific type of food, ones that are high in carbohydrates, sugars, and fats.

Typically cakes, chips, cookies, etc. When eating because of emotional hunger, it's much more difficult to stop, and generally, you continue eating even after becoming full.

Emotional hunger can happen suddenly and without warning. You could be going about your day, feeling completely normal, and all of a sudden start craving cake. Unlike real hunger, you can't think of anything else except you're craving, and have this strong need to fulfil it right away. While you're eating, you feel happy and comforted; eating makes the bad feelings go away. However, once you've eaten, you have this feeling of guilt or shame. You know what you ate is bad for you, but you still couldn't help yourself. You feel horrible and start feeling those negative thoughts again. But instead of feeling what you felt before, you feel even more stressed, and you're not sure how to process it or get rid of it.

Chapter 13: Finding Other Activities to Replace Emotional Eating

WHEN YOU FIGURE OUT what your triggers are and understand why you're emotionally eating, it's essential to find various things that can replace the overeating. The biggest thing to take into consideration is that emotional eating is for comfort. So it makes sense that you replace emotional eating with something that is also a comfort to you. If it doesn't comfort you on the same level, then you'll just go back to eating emotionally.

There are many different things you can do; you just have to find what works best for you. You also have to be realistic about it. Are you the type of person that likes going out of their way for something? Do you like driving a little bit before eating? Do you like trying new restaurants? If you do, replace the restaurant with a different sort of store. Try going to thrift stores, or art studios. A place that you can drive to, but it's still healthy and you won't overeat.

Most people use food to replace comfort because it's convenient and quick, so it's best to find a comfort that reflects the same thing. Figure out something that's easy and within reach. The most important thing is to pick something that works for you. You might have a friend who loves to paint, but it might not necessarily be the right activity for you.

Here are some good examples you can try:

- **Go for a walk**
- **Read a book**
- **Call a friend**

Social Media (*this one might seem silly but spending time on a forum or your social media page will distract you from eating emotionally! Plus, you can talk with international friends, which can also be a great distraction. You can even find an online group for emotional eaters and talk with people who understand what you're going through.*)

Make a cup of tea

Take a nap (*it's possible you're feeling exhausted, so think that eating something sugary will help perk you up. And while that's technically true, it's not very healthy. Even if it's in the evening, a 20-minute power nap can do wonders for your energy.*)

- **Crosswords/Puzzles**
- **Video Games**

Cook (*Replace the junk food with healthy, home-cooked meals. You can spend time prepping, putting together recipes, even shopping at the store. Make sure to buy just what's on your list, so you don't accidentally relapse.*)

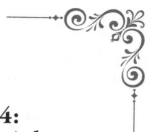

Chapter 14:
Questions to Ask
Yourself Before You
Eat Something

IT'S A GREAT IDEA TO stop a moment before actually eating. It's an empowering way to talk to yourself, and make sure what you're doing is actually good for you. You've heard the saying "Your body is a temple", so why not treat it as such?

Here are some questions to ask yourself before eating:

If I eat this, how will it make me feel in an hour?

Maybe you're eating a regular meal, and you'll be completely fine in an hour. But perhaps you're thinking of eating an entire cake (don't worry, we've all been there!). How will eating that cake make you feel? Are you fat, bloated, sick, possibly feeling good but in a terrible way? Then move on to something else!

Am I going to regret this?

You've successfully stayed away from fries for months. It's an amazing feeling and one that you're proud of, but man, those fries look so good. If you eat them, will you regret it? Of course, you will; you've broken your winning streak, and with the re-introduction of these fries, you'll soon start telling yourself that you'll start not eating them again tomorrow. Or the next day, or the next day, until months from now when you realize that you've eaten fries every day.

Am I eating this just because my friends are and it's fun?

Eating can be very social, and it's easy to get caught up in how much fun you're having with your friends. If you're eating something just because it's fun, you won't be feeling so happy about it afterwards. Do you really want to put yourself through that emotional upheaval?

Am I eating just because I'm bored?

What if you did something else for a bit? Are you still hungry, or was it just because you were bored? Try working on a hobby, or talking with a friend, and see if you're no longer hungry.

Am I thirsty?

Hunger pains are often mistaken for thirst, so it's entirely possible that you're just in need of water! Drink a glass of water first. If you're full, then you weren't really hungry. Besides, drinking more water is always a good practice to get into anyway.

What exactly is this doing to my body?

This is a great question to ask, regardless of when or what you're eating. You wouldn't feed chocolate to a dog, so why would you be putting bad things in your own body? And while you might not have an immediate allergic reaction like a dog would with chocolate, it's still unhealthy in the long-term sense.

Chapter 15: Why You Should Seek Therapy for Emotional Eating

WHAT HAPPENS WHEN YOU get a cold? You try several over the counter medications, but the cold just won't go away. So you decide to bite the bullet and just go into a clinic. They prescribe some stronger stuff, and your cold is gone within days. People even insist you see a doctor; after all, they're worried about your health, and possibly themselves getting sick. What about when you get a broken bone? People aren't going to say things like "Can't you just feel better?" or "It's all in your head". They're going to make sure you see a doctor and understand that you might be a little less capable the next few weeks.

So why don't we do the same thing when it comes to our mental and emotional health? If we see a doctor when our bodies are sick, then why don't we see one when our minds aren't feeling well?

There's definitely a stigma when it comes to therapy. It's thought that only people who have mental disorders, like schizophrenia, are the ones to seek psychological help.

However, therapy can be used for many different things and is very beneficial when dealing with mental or emotional issues.

Cognitive Behavior Therapy is a very effective therapy that can help someone learn to deal with their emotional eating. How it works is within the title itself; it's a form of therapy that changes your way of thinking. It's done in a non-intrusive manner and is focused mainly on how to change the way you specifically think about things.

A therapist will go over your expectations in the beginning and put forth a positive vibe to ensure full cooperation. It has to be something you actually want, or else it won't work, and you'll be disappointed with the results.

The cognitive part of it involves paying nonjudgmental attention to what and how you're thinking at the present moment. It involves looking inward and taking a reflection of what you're thinking, helping to increase your awareness of your emotions, and learning how to separate emotions from hunger.

There's a behaviour modification part of it as well. You learn techniques to replace eating with other activities, how to specifically stop emotional eating, and how to deal with strong emotions in a different manner.

There's also the possibility that your stress stems from another source, and emotional eating is used to cover it up. We all deal with normal daily stress, but Post-Traumatic Stress Disorder is a real possibility. There might have been a traumatic moment in your past, and therapy is the only real way of figuring out what it was and how to stop it from affecting you negatively. There's also the risk of clinical depression, anxiety disorders, or emotional eating turning into a more serious eating disorder.

It's very important to get professional help. Just because we can't do it ourselves, doesn't mean we have to do it alone.

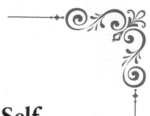

Chapter 16: Self-care Tips to Manage Emotional Eating

EMOTIONAL EATING IS very difficult to manage and can be a strain on us, both physically and mentally. There's no one answer when trying to figure it out; you just have to do what works best for you.

Here are some self-care tips to manage your emotional eating:

Don't be hard on yourself:

Food is a form of comfort, and sometimes we just need something to comfort us. Yes, it's not healthy to emotionally eat. But one of the worst things you can do is blame yourself or feel bad about yourself after eating. There are different ways you can manage it and making yourself feel ashamed isn't one of them.

Be Mindful of Your Decision:

If you go in knowing that you're about to eat that piece of cake because you're feeling upset, then you're more likely not to eat as much. Sit and think while you're eating, think about each bite while you're chewing it. Yes, you're feeling upset, and yes, you're eating because you need the comfort. Maybe just a few bites will work instead of the whole piece? Reevaluate your feelings after a few bites and see how you're feeling. If you're no longer feeling upset, then there's no need to eat anymore.

Focus on Another Sense:

The main reason we go to food for comfort is that it tastes really good. We're stimulating our taste buds! So what about our other senses? Try focusing on one of those instead and see what happens. Look at pretty pictures, listen to different sounds. Try something unusual, something that will help you to focus on things other than food. There are videos called ASMR - Autonomous Sensory Meridian Response. Some have people that speak very softly and gently into a microphone; some create loud sounds from quiet ones. Activities like making raindrops sound much louder than they are, or fabric rubbing together. Watching these is a great way to stimulate your ears and will help you focus on something other than your taste buds. You could also light a candle or wrap yourself up in a warm blanket. Doing this will give you a certain level of comfort and will replace that feeling you get from eating.

Speak Like Your Royalty:

You will definitely feel silly doing this! But start talking to yourself in the 3rd person. Instead of saying, "I'm a failure" or "I never do anything right", try using your name - "Ashley is a failure" or "Ashley never does anything right". Saying things like that out loud puts things into perspective. It's almost as if you're speaking about someone else, and most people don't talk that way about others. Would you say those things about your parents? What about your children? Counter those by peppering in compliments too! Say things like "Ashley is looking great today", or something a lot more specific - "This shirt Ashley is wearing really makes her eyes pop". Giving yourselves compliments in the 3rd person will seem ridiculous! But one of the reasons for emotional eating is due to self-destructive tendencies, so by telling yourself compliments, you'll start feeling better about yourself.

Start a new 'getting home from work' habit:

Another great trick is trying something new once you get home from work. Most of us get home and go straight for the food. It's been a long day at work, and curling up on the couch with a pizza sounds so good, right? Instead of going straight to the fridge though, begin a new non-food habit. As soon as you get through the door, try playing with your pet, looking out a window, or do a few stretches. It doesn't have to be an exercise. You could even watch a YouTube video! Just make it a habit, and soon you'll be doing that instead of going for the junk food. Having this little transition time between work and dinner will help put things into perspective. You'll be able to reflect, decompress, and center yourself. This will, in turn, help you to make better eating choices.

Press reset:

An interesting trick you can use is to reset your body. Emotional eaters tend to get caught up in their minds and end up only being able to focus on food. Using little things to jolt yourself out of this mindset can actually work! Try holding a piece of ice, running your hands under cold or hot water, or even biting into a lemon, lime, or grapefruit. All these things give your body a jolt and force it to wake up from the current thoughts you're having. It's a sort of mind reset, and a great way to refocus your thoughts on something other than food.

Chapter 17: How Mindful Eating Can Help

MINDFUL EATING IS EXACTLY what the name implies - being mindful of what you're eating! It allows you to be a little more attentive to what's going on at the moment, which helps with binging and overeating. It slows everything down and gets you out of automatic food habits. It also allows for better management of your emotions. It allows you to tolerate your emotions, without covering them up with food. Similar to Cognitive Behavior Therapy, it changes the way you think. It helps redirect your thoughts to a more positive experience when eating.

Mindful eating also helps your body recognize cues of when to stop eating. One of the major issues with emotional eating is not stopping when you're full. You end up overeating and feeling terrible because of it. Using mindful eating, you can focus on how your body is feeling, and learning when actually to stop eating.

It can be split up into 5 different actions that you take while you're eating or thinking about eating something:

1. **Observe.** What exactly is your body doing at the

moment? Is your stomach actually growling? Are you feeling tired, fatigued, stressed, satisfied, full, or empty? Are you hungry, or just compensating for a different feeling?

1. **Be in the moment.** If you are eating, just be doing that. Turn off the TV, step away from your phone. Be fully present while eating, which allows you to focus on your food and just that.

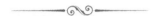

1. **Aware.** Be aware when eating. Are you thinking and tasting your food, or just going through the motions?

1. **Savor.** Notice the texture of your food. What spices do you taste? What does it smell like? Is it crunchy or smooth?

1. **Non-judgment.** Don't be harsh with yourself! Speak to yourself compassionately and mindfully. Take notice of when guild and "should" sentences pop into your mind.

IF YOU'RE NOT READY to start mindful eating with your food, you can always try it out on other things first. Start by being mentally present during a moment. Most of us tend to multitask; we're on our phones when talking with someone, etc. So, try putting down your phone during a conversation, or not getting on your phone during an elevator ride. If you're waiting on someone, try just looking around and observe what's around you. It's a great way to "train" yourself to be mindful while eating!

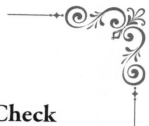

Chapter 18: Check Your Hunger Scale

WHAT EXACTLY IS THE Hunger Scale? It's not an actual physical scale that you step on, but rather a numbered one that you can use to judge how hungry you really are.

It's important to take a step back and understand if you're actually hungry or just feeling like you could eat a bite or two. With emotional eating, it can be very easy to eat a whole meal, even though you aren't hungry. So using the hunger scale is a very effective way to help with that.

Think about it like this: Babies and small children don't just keep eating and eating. They're able to stop once they're full. This means we're born with the ability to feel fullness. Yet, emotional eaters tend to feel empty due to emotional issues, so try to fill up that emptiness with food.

Using the hunger scale which ranges 1-10, we can train ourselves to relearn that feeling of fullness:

1 - Empty - Put food in my mouth right now or I'm going to kill somebody! Has the feeling of dizziness and lightheadedness. I'll take everything on the menu. A general feeling of hunger.

2 - Really Hungry - Feeling dizzy, poor concentration, mood swings, energy levels are down. Give me food or I'm going to crash soon.

3 - Hungry - The normal amount of hungry before eating a meal. Need to eat soon, or else I'm going to get very unpleasant.

4 - Slightly Hungry - Might be thinking about my next meal, but I don't have to eat right away. I can wait a bit, it's no big deal.

5 - Neutral - Neither hungry nor empty. I'm completely fine, not thinking about food at all.

6 - Somewhat Satisfied - I could eat a little more of my meal. If I stop now, then I'll probably be hungry again in a couple hours.

7 - Satisfied - I don't actually have to eat any more, I'm feeling perfectly satisfied. I might have a few more bites because the food is yummy, but it's not necessary.

8 - Full - I probably shouldn't have had those extra few bites, what was I thinking? Good thing I'm wearing yoga pants!

9 - Uncomfortable - I really shouldn't have eaten all of that. I'm feeling way too full and am zoning out from everyone's conversations. I even feel slightly nauseated.

10 - Thanksgiving Full - I'm a beached whale, I'm literally bursting out of my pants. The only relief I feel is curling up on the cool tile floor and hoping I don't pass out. The only acceptable solution is going into a coma and focusing all my energy into digesting.

So how do you use the hunger scale? It's a lot to think about and deal with while also trying to figure out what to eat. The best thing you can do is take it one step at a time.

First, figure out exactly where you rank before eating anything. Have you not eaten since dinner yesterday? Or did you just eat an hour ago, and are simply feeling bored? If you within the 1 - 2 range, be extra cautious when eating. When you're hungry to that extent, it's very easy to overeat. You could jump from a 1 to a 9 in one meal, which would even possibly make you sick! This is where Mindful Eating comes in handy. Go through the actions of mindful eating when you're feeling this hungry, and it'll help you to slow down enough that you won't accidentally overeat.

Once you're halfway through your meal, stop and rank yourself again. Are you still hungry or are you feeling satisfied? The last thing you want to do is eat on autopilot, especially if you started out in the 1 - 2 range of the hunger scale. If you're reaching the 7 - 8 range, stop. If food remains on your plate, ask for a to-go container, or pack up the leftovers yourself. If you're the type of person that hates leftovers, and just can't make yourself eat them, then just throw away the food. It might seem like a waste, and you might even feel guilty for doing it, but the guilt of throwing away food is much better than the guilt and shame of overeating.

If you decide to continue your meal, rank yourself again once you've finished. If you're feeling a good level of satisfied, then the portions were correct, and you didn't overeat. Awesome job! If you're feeling overly full, then ask yourself why you didn't stop eating before. Maybe the food was just too tasty, maybe you were too hungry when you started, or perhaps you didn't want to waste it. Whichever the reason, don't feel guilty for letting it happen. Just recognize and understand why it happened, which will help you to prevent it in the future.

Before actually using it, you have to make sure your hunger scale is accurately working. If you've been trying to diet and it's not sticking, or if you've been counting calories for a while, it's possible that your body will be out of sync with real hunger and fullness. If you've started to skip breakfast, and you're starving by the time lunch rolls around, then it's obvious what the issue is. The best way to "recalibrate" your hunger scale is eating well-proportioned meals, typically about 4 to 5 hours apart.

Once you get into the normal pattern of eating, it'll be easier to determine where you fall on the hunger scale for each meal.

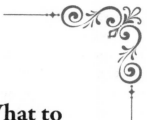

Chapter 19: What to Do Before You Eat Something

IT CAN BE DIFFICULT to stop yourself from eating something. You're feeling stressed, bored, even happy, and the next thing you know is that you have a plate of food. It almost seems to happen automatically, so how do you stop something like that from happening?

Here are a few tips and tricks you can try before actually eating something:

Back it up now y'all

Take a step back. Literally, if you have too! Let's say you just got home from work and find yourself heading straight into the kitchen. Take a step back, and just pause for a moment. Sometimes that pause is all we need to realize that we're not hungry, but just going through the motions of a habit. What if you're out with friends? You can't exactly stand up from the table and step back, not when other customers and waiters are running around. So instead of automatically getting dessert when your waiter asks if you want it, take a breath and pause. We're a society of instant gratification and having that extra pause will help you to decide if you really need the extra food.

Rehydrate

Our bodies are wired a little oddly, and sometimes it's easy to mistake thirst for hunger pains. It's entirely possible that you're not actually hungry, but thirsty instead. So drink a glass of water first, before eating anything.

It's a good practice to have anyway; it's essential to get 8 cups of water a day. So, getting into the habit of drinking a glass before eating anything is probably smart. And it's not just for meals! Even drinking water before snacks is good because it stops you from overeating when you're not even actually hungry. If you're just not into water (and some people aren't!), then try making a cup of tea instead. The simple act of making one can refocus your thoughts, and you end up not thinking about food.

Phone a friend

Maybe what you're looking for isn't food, but comfort. Perhaps you had a hard day at work, and all you want is a little comfort. Food makes the most sense in your mind; it's right there in front of you, and you can get to it right away. And sometimes it can be weirdly tricky talking with friends on the phone. But instead of reaching for those chips, try reaching for your phone instead. Even just that simple action will help deter you from emotionally eating. And since you already have your phone in hand, it makes sense just to make a quick call to a friend or loved one. It doesn't have to be specific conversation either; just ask them how their day was and tell them about your day in return. This is very cathartic too! Telling someone about your day can help relieve stress, which will prevent you from overeating.

Dear Diary

Write it down! It doesn't matter what you write; what your day was like, a weird thing you saw on the bus today, the conversation you had with your boss. As long as you're writing things down and getting your thoughts out. It helps you to de-stress and prevents you from overeating due to that stress; it's along the same lines as phoning a friend. In addition, writing even a few sentences will help you to gather your thoughts, reflect inwards, and decide if you're starving or using food to cover something else you're feeling. If you don't like writing, then try drawing something. It doesn't have to be considered "art"; you can doodle a few scribbles. The act of writing/drawing helps get your energy and emotions out in a much healthier way than eating.

Chapter 20: How Intuitive Eating Can Help You

INTUITIVE EATING IS all about bringing it back to basics. Babies and children have that ability to stop eating when they feel full. Sometimes, they don't even eat at all because they're not hungry! But as we grow up, we're told to finish everything on our plate, and dessert is used as a bribe. We feel guilty when eating specific foods because we're told some foods are better for us than others. As we get older, we start trying different diets and doing things like counting calories. Sometimes that works, but sometimes it doesn't. And do you want to live the rest of your life continually counting calories?

Intuitive eating doesn't rely on the "normal" fad diets but is more about listening to your body. Your body will tell you when you're hungry when you're craving a little sweet.

Intuitive eating rulebook:

1. The first thing you need to do when using intuitive eating is to throw out the diet handbook. Forget all the different things you've read about diets! It's a system to set you up for failure, and definitely succeeds in that fact! All that diets do is to make you feel bad about yourself.

2. Being hungry is ok! What happens when you skip a meal? You just get hungrier later, until you end up binge eating your next meal. This is what you're trying to stay away from. If you're hungry, then eat! Even if it's at a weird time. And it doesn't have to be a huge meal - even just a little snack will work. As long as you're satisfying your bodies need for hunger.

3. One huge thing that people deal with when being an emotional eater is continuing to eat even though they're full because they're not satisfied. Let's say you're hungry and craving something. You want something sweet but know it's unhealthy, so you eat a sandwich instead. But you haven't satisfied that sweet craving, so you eat the sandwich, and just keep eating because you aren't satisfied. All of a sudden, you realize that you've eaten three sandwiches! But if you had just eaten something like a piece of chocolate, then you would've felt satisfied and wouldn't have overeaten. Sometimes it's better to satisfy your craving because there are fewer repercussions. One little piece of chocolate is definitely better than three sandwiches.

4. Get in touch with your feelings! When you're eating, pause for a minute halfway. Do you feel full? Sometimes we feel like we have to keep eating, especially when with other people. But it's ok to stop, especially when we're full. Think about it like this - if you stop halfway, you can box up the leftovers to take home. Then you get to eat this amazing meal again! And remember that being healthy doesn't mean you eat perfectly all the time. It's ok to eat foods that make you feel better, but it's all about proportions and consistency. If you have one unhealthy thing, it won't cause weight gain. The problems start only when you eat that one unhealthy thing over and over again.

5. What about exercise? It's definitely a way to get healthy, but it has to be something you like doing. If you can't stand jogging and only do it as a way to be healthy, it's not something you'll stick with. Find something you really like that gets you moving. Maybe take a dance class or join a hiking group. If it's something you love, then it won't feel like work to you.

6. Quiet those inner thoughts! You know the ones - "This meal is good for me because it's a salad", "I'm eating bad today because I had carbs". These are thoughts that have been ingrained in us from various diets that make it impossible to view eating as normal. Some salads are actually bad for us, and it won't kill you to eat carbs. So tell those pesky thoughts to shut up, and you just enjoy your meal.

7. Respect! Aretha Franklin might have been talking about demanding respect from her man, but the same concept applies to you and your own body. Don't be too hard on yourself! Learn to respect how your body is at the moment. What happens when we put ourselves down? We start feeling bad, and the only way to feel better is by eating. But then we feel even worse because we just binge eat! It's a vicious loop and needs to stop. By truly accepting who we are and what we look like, we can help ourselves in the long run.

Intuitive Eating takes the ideas of Mindful Eating one step further. Mindful eating is about understanding your feelings when it comes to eating and respecting your own inner choices. Intuitive eating denies the diet mentality and helps you to respect your body, no matter what size and shape you are. Using both together is a fantastic way to help cope with emotional eating.

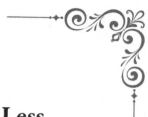

Chapter 21: Less Obvious Signs You Are an Emotional Eater

WE COVERED ALL THE usual signs that you're an emotional eater - you eat when stressed, upset, happy, etc. You eat to feel comfort, or you even eat just because you can't stop thinking about food. What about the less obvious signs? What if you're not the type of person to constantly think about food? How are you supposed to know if you're an emotional eater or not?

Here are some not-so-obvious signs that you're an emotional eater:

1. Fear of missing out. We've all seen it - a friend or family member posting on social media about doing something that looks super fun. And of course, the first thought we have is why they didn't invite us or that what they're doing seems amazing and you wish you were doing it too. It's called "fear of missing out" and can also be applied to food. Maybe you follow a foodie on Instagram; someone that posts all the time about this amazing new food they found around town. You realize you absolutely have to have it and can't focus on anything else until you eat whatever they had. Or maybe you're with a friend who happens to be eating something really yummy. And even though you're not hungry, you still want to snatch that yummy treat out of their hands and scarf it down. Or all your friends are on their third drink of the night, and it seems like they're having a much better time than you. Maybe if you have a third drink, then you'll feel whatever happiness and good feelings they're experiencing.

2. You hide what you eat. You're happy that your roommate or another important person is working late! Not because you get some much needed alone time, but because you can break out your secret stash of cookies and eat as many as you want without them finding out. After all, it would be so embarrassing if they found out how much you actually eat, right? We hide our food because we have this belief that something is wrong with us, and if people honestly *really* knew what was going on, then they won't love us.

3. Procrastinate life. "I'll start dating once I get in shape". "I can't go on this trip because I'm just too overweight". "Maybe once I'm in shape, then I'll start doing fun things". Emotional eaters overeat, which in turn develops a bad relationship with their bodies. These bad feelings cause even more eating because of that need for comfort, which creates a loop of eating and feelings. But it also causes you to put your life on hold, with no end in sight. You keep putting things off until you're "healthy", thinking it makes more sense to wait. But how long are you supposed to wait? You only have a limited time on this world; do you want to spend most of it thinking about things you want to do instead of just doing it? It's a vicious trap and one that's very difficult to get out of.

4. **Addiction.** Sugars are addictive. It's actually scientifically a fact; sugar releases a chemical called 'dopamine', which in turn makes us feel happy. It's entirely possible you have an addiction to sugar and don't even know it! Maybe you constantly chew gum that's high in sugar. Maybe you need to have a donut every morning. Maybe you need to add a lot of sugar to your coffee. What makes you an emotional eater is the fact that you need sugar to feel happy, instead of doing something else instead. It's hard to change a habit, even more so when it's one that makes you feel a sense of happiness. The key is finding something that also makes you feel happy but in a much healthier way.

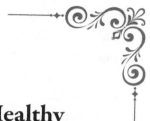

Chapter 22: Healthy Ways to Manage Your Stress

THIS IS PROBABLY GOING to be one of the most difficult things you change about yourself. It's extremely hard to change a habit and requires a lot of willpower and determination. However, if you choose the right technique for you, then it will be so much easier! You have to find something that works with your personality and daily routine. Otherwise it'll be a "habit" that doesn't last very long.

1. Avoid caffeine, alcohol, and nicotine

This one is probably the most difficult option!! All of these are addictive, and coffee tends to be a must-have with most people. If you like having a cup or three every morning, it will be very hard to stop. Luckily, there are little tricks you can use to help! Switching to decaf will certainly help. You still get the placebo of having coffee in the mornings, but without dealing with high stress levels the rest of the day. You can also switch to water, herbal teas, or naturally diluted juice.

2. Sleep more!

Sleep is very important when managing stress. Getting a good night's rest helps us to feel more relaxed and just overall better the next day. It can be hard to truly fall asleep though. Sometimes we stress so much about our lives that we stay up for hours. The key to this is to be as relaxed as possible before bedtime. Avoid drinking and eating things you know will make you stressed, like alcohol and caffeine. Read a book or take a calming bath right before bed to help relax your mind and body. It also helps tremendously to go to bed around the same time each night. Your body and mind get into the habit, which helps with a consistent night sleep.

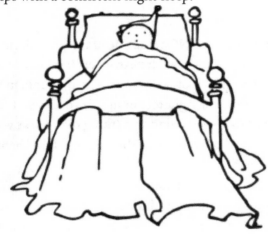

3. Physical Activity

You don't have to run a marathon! The simple act of simply taking a walk before bedtime can help reduce stress. Stress produces adrenaline, which triggers the feeling of "fight or flight". But when we don't actually fight or flight, our bodies feel even more stressed because they're expecting to do something and that thing isn't happening. Physical activity can trick the body and mind and restore them to a much more relaxed state. Anytime you feel stressed or tense, do some physical activity. Either go for a short walk or do some stretches. Try and do something every day! This can be before or after work, or even during your lunch break. Soon you'll get into the habit of exercising, which will in return make you feel healthier and happier.

4. Try relaxation techniques.

Sometimes we have to teach ourselves to relax. Maybe it's something you've never learned or got out of the habit of doing. Whatever the reason is, you have to be able to choose the right technique that works for you, otherwise you won't keep up with it and the stress will just come back. And don't worry if it's difficult at first; relaxation is a skill that needs to be learned and practiced.

Some different relaxation techniques you can try:

➡ You can try lying on your back in a dark room and focusing on breathing in and out. Let your entire body relax, from the top of your head to your toes. It almost feels like you're letting your body sink into the ground, one muscle at a time.

➡ Stand up straight and clench your body while tightening your muscles and hunching over. While doing this, just breathe in through your nose. Hold this position and count to five. After you've reached five, breathe back out through your nose and start relaxing your body. You'll start to feel as if a huge weight has been lifted off of you, which will help you to feel more relaxed.

➡ You can also try self-hypnosis. Which does sound odd, but don't worry - you won't start clucking like a chicken! It's something that's easy and can be done anywhere, from sitting at your desk to sitting in your car. The main idea of it is to focus on one word or phrase that conveys a positive meaning to you.

Words like "love", "calm", and "peace" work really well. Or even phrases like "grant me serenity" or "I am calm" work as well. Focus on your mantra and repeat it until you feel calm. You might have random thoughts pop up; acknowledge and disregard them, then return to your mantra. Repeat whenever you feel stressed or tense.

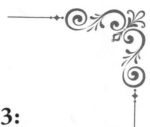

Chapter 23:
Beginner Tips for
Meditating

MEDITATION CAN BE A great way to calm your mind, reduce stress, and focus on your inner thoughts. It can help you learn to control your emotions and redirect your feelings into something other than eating. It can seem difficult to learn; most people find it difficult to sit for hours and think about nothing. It's a skill and habit that needs to be learned, which takes dedication and practice. But it's worth it! Not only does it help with feeling stressed, but meditation can also help you to understand who you are as a person, and how your mind works. It gives you a certain type of freedom and awareness.

It is not a very easy habit to get into, but there are ways! The key is to start small and work your way up.

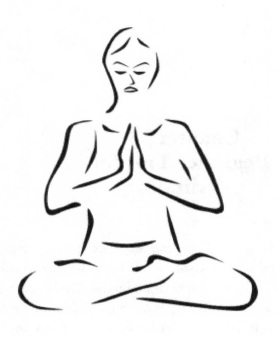

Here are some tips and tricks you can use to help focus your thoughts and learn how to meditate successfully.

1. First thing.

Try meditating first thing in the morning. Literally first thing! You can even meditate in your bed before getting out, which sounds really cozy and nice. Try setting an alarm or write a note somewhere; having that extra reminder will help you to remember and stay on track.

2. Two minutes

Meditate for just two minutes. Doesn't sound too bad, right? It's not that long, and easy enough to work into a busy schedule! Start with two minutes the first week, then, increase it by another two minutes each week. So week 1 is 2 minutes, week 2 is 4 minutes, week 3 is 6 minutes, etc. You'll be up to 30 minutes in a few months, which is enough time to form a habit. Pretty soon you won't feel normal unless you start your day with meditation!

3. Just do it!

Don't think about all the little details, especially at first. Instead of thinking about where you're sitting, where you're facing, what you're sitting in, just sit down and start. It's not for that long, especially at first since you're only doing it for two minutes. Once you've upped your time, you can worry about being a little more comfortable. But in the beginning, just sit and meditate.

4. Counting breaths

It can be hard to concentrate, especially when first learning how to meditate. Your mind will wander and you will start thinking about other things. These can be about how your nose is itchy, or what you're doing that day. An easy way to refocus is by counting your breaths. Pay close attention to what your breathing is doing, about how it's filling your lungs and then leaving your body. Focus on each breath and count them one by one. Once you've reached ten, start over at one and keep counting to ten. It's completely normal to not feel focused and get frustrated with yourself. If that happens, just smile and start over counting your breaths.

5. Love yourself

You'll get many different thoughts and feelings pop up when meditating. And that's ok! Accept the thought and move on. Realize that your thoughts are a part of you and look at them in a friendly manner. One of the most significant concerns you might think about is that you're not meditating correctly. There's no wrong way to meditate, and you have to do what feels right for you. Replace any negative thoughts with positive ones and remember to be happy that you have started something as tricky as meditating!

6. Blank space

Many people think meditating is all about clearing the mind of all thoughts. Sometimes this does happen, but it's actually incredibly difficult to clear your mind in this manner. It's normal to have thoughts, and difficult to stop them. If random thoughts do pop up, try to refocus your attention by counting your breaths or something similar.

Or you can even try the opposite! When a thought or feeling comes along, try staying with it for a while. Maybe you're feeling stressed, but you don't know why. And as you're sitting there meditating, that feeling of stress comes along again. Instead of dismissing it, accept it and let it stay. Acknowledge that it's there. Accepting it will allow you to let it go that much easier later on. Sometimes we need to deal with our stress or other strong feelings head-on in order to actually work through them.

7. Scan your body

Meditation is a great way to get to know and understand yourself. As you're sitting there, what are you feeling? How are you feeling? Start at the soles of the feet and work your way up. Take it one step at a time, and really focus on each part of your body. Your body deserves your attention, and it will help you to feel so much better at the end.

8. Other senses

After you've focused on counting breaths for a couple of weeks, try focusing on your other senses. What sounds do you hear around you? What do you smell? Maybe you've decided to meditate in your backyard, which has many sounds and smells to focus on. Even try to notice the energy around you. What are those birds doing? Can you feel the wind blowing on your face? Honing in on other things besides your breath can help you to focus mentally and gives your mind a break from the daily stresses you encounter.

9. Commit

Really give meditation a go. Don't just say you'll try it for a couple of weeks, but if you don't see any results, then you're stopping. Meditation is a subtle skill that takes time to learn, and you might not know if it's working for a while. Any habit takes at least a month to form, so at the very least, give yourself about a month and see how you feel after.

10. Anywhere, anytime

Meditation is something you can actually do anywhere. If you're running late in the morning, wait until you get to your office. You can just sit in your office chair for a couple of minutes, counting your breaths and focusing on the sounds around you. Or you can go to the park during your lunch break. You can even try it as you're walking! Instead of thinking about what you're doing the rest of your day or that annoying phone call you had, think about what you hear around you. Do you listen to lots of cars or signs of traffic? What do you see? Focus on your senses, which will help stop you thinking about things that have been stressing you.

11. Accountability

Sometimes it helps to have an accountability buddy or partner; someone you can call about your meditation. Set something up with a friend - maybe you can call them before you start or after. Even sending a text can help! All you can to do is send a message stating you're about to begin your meditation, and you're more likely actually to do it. Have your friend ask you how it went, which will help you to keep up with it until it's become a habit.

12. Community

Sometimes having a community of like-minded peers can be beneficial. There are meditation classes you can join or groups you can meet up with. Most Buddhist and Tibetan temples allow anyone to participate in their meditation. It might actually be a fantastic experience! Instead of meditating at home, surrounded by distractions, you can meditate with Buddhist monks. Not only are you with people who understand the benefits of meditation, but you're also surroundings are ideal for relaxation and will have a calming effect on you.

13. Guides

Some people like having a step-by-step guide to follow. Instead of just jumping right in and hoping for the best, try looking up a guide you can refer to. Guides can be helpful and provide various tips and rules that you can try.

14. Befriend yourself

This one might seem a little trivial but, become your own friend. Don't be too harsh on yourself! You're learning a new skill and habit, which takes time to develop. Keep a friendly attitude instead of one with criticism. If you're teaching someone something new, do you constantly critique or give encouragement? Remember to give yourself a little love.

15. Smile when you're done!

You have just accomplished something amazing! Even if it was only for two minutes, you had time to yourself, gave a full commitment, got to know yourself, and took the time to become friends with yourself. You were able to focus on your inner self, and step away from the stress. If that doesn't deserve a smile, then what does? Also, as an added bonus - the act of smiling can actually cause you to feel happier! So not only did you just accomplish something great, you made yourself feel happy about it. Think about how incredible it would be to feel this way every day!

Chapter 24: How to Recover From an Emotional Eating Binge

WE'VE ALL BEEN THERE. It's been a day full of stress, from both your professional life and personal one. The last thing you want to do is go home and cook, so you decide just to forget it and binge out on junk food. And should it not be so? It makes you feel better, it makes your troubles seem to disappear, and it allows you to go into an almost daze which helps you to forget about the stress you've just experienced. But then it happens. The aftermath: The realisation of what you've just done.

"Why do I do this to myself?"

"Why am I like this?"

"What's wrong with me?"

The realization that while you felt better for a little bit, now you're feeling even worse than before. What do you do know? How could you possibly recover from something like this?

The first thing you do is go easy on yourself. Don't beat yourself up for a mistake. The worst feelings happen after emotionally binge eating; shame, hopelessness, anger. You feel like you just destroyed yourself, and that you blew it. That you've tried so hard to be good with food, but you failed again. Instead of being angry at yourself, tell yourself this key phrase:

It Happens

Binge eating happens. It's part of being an emotional eater, and it's going to happen! But the thing to remember is that recovery from binge eating isn't about never binging again. It's about eating less and less, at a less frequent rate. As you binge eat less frequently, you replace it with other, much more healthy, things.

The key is to get past the guilt. It's done, it happened, and you need to move past it.

The best way to get past it is by becoming something of a detective. Figure out why it happened. Were you hungry? Upset? Stressed? Why did you decide to binge eat now, after not doing it for the past two weeks? Once you recognize the issue, it'll be that much easier to prevent it from happening again.

Once you've figured out why it's happened, get back to your usual routine. It's so very easy just to say 'forget it', and just let loose since you've already binged. What's one more day of binge eating if you've already done it? But getting back into your routine can help things feel more normal, which in turn makes it less likely that you'll binge out again.

One very vital thing to remember is that **you're not alone.** It can be really difficult to reach out to family and friends after binge eating. Emotional eating is associated with shame, and it can feel embarrassing to admit that you're an emotional eater. But in having someone to talk to about it can be beneficial! You have the option of communicating with family and friends about it, but some people are too embarrassed to do even that.

Fortunately, there are options that you can explore. Online groups are a great way to connect with people who understand what you're going through. You can hold each other accountable and commiserate together when one of you slips up. It's a great way to feel not as ashamed and have others in your life that can help you through the strong negative feelings you experience.

Another option is speaking to a professional. Either a psychologist or your doctor can help. Emotional eating is a disorder and lately has started to be recognized as one officially. A doctor can help keep you on track, and a psychologist makes for a great sounding board.

Sometimes it's helpful to have an actual list you can follow after binge eating. What follows are some ideas you can implement after an emotional eating binge episode. You can do all of them, or just one. What's important is to find out what works best for you and stick with it!

1. **Forgive yourself.** Remember that things happen, and it's not your fault. Don't be too hard on yourself.

1. **Keep the next meals clean and healthy.** Don't keep binge eating the rest of the day. Accept that it happened and move on to healthier foods for your next meals.
2. **Go for a walk.** Getting up and moving around can help digestion and help overcome that general "blah" feeling. Plus, exercising releases endorphins, which puts you in a good mood!

1. **Don't starve yourself in retaliation.** Don't go without food for the rest of the day. You might think it's better since you ate so much, but it actually makes things worse. You'll end up super hungry, which can lead to more binge eating.
2. **Forget that the scale exists.** Don't focus on weighing yourself! Binge eating leads to feelings of shame and regret and weighing yourself immediately after will only emphasize those feelings.
3. **Hydrate!** Drinking water aids in digestion and helps to flush out any excess salt you may have consumed. It's also really good for supporting a healthy metabolism and makes it less likely you'll binge eat another meal.
4. **Get enough sleep.** It seems counter-productive to sleep after eating a big meal. Wouldn't it make more sense to exercise instead? But getting enough sleep can actually help with food restraint. You'll feel less tired, less stressed, and less likely to binge eat.

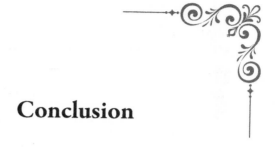

Conclusion

THANK YOU FOR MAKING it through to the end of *Emotional Eating*! I sincerely hope it was informative and able to provide you with all of the tools you need to achieve your goals.

It takes a lot of work to overcome being an emotional eater. It takes dedication, will-power, forgiveness, self-love, and hope. It means forming healthy habits.

Whether you journal, meditate, join an online community, or knit, just remember that it isn't something that happens overnight. You need patience and the right information to help see you through.

While you need this information, it can seem like a lot, and be very overwhelming at first. Just start with a few simple questions: Are you an emotional eater? Are you exhibiting the right signs? What are your triggers?

Once you understand a little more about emotional eating, the next step is to figure out how to help yourself in ways that work best for you.

This book covers many different tips and tricks you can practice and use to help counter the effects of emotional eating. Maybe you love writing things down, so journaling works best for you. Perhaps you prefer meditation or exercise. Maybe you love dancing, so what works best for you are throwing yourself a dance party instead of a binging session.

The most important thing is to remember self-care. Never put yourself down and remember that you are only human. It's ok to mess up, as long as you pick yourself back up and move forward.

The key to this is forming healthy habits and keeping up with them. Once you start doing that, then you're on the right track for eating healthier and losing weight.

And remember:-

Be proud! You've accomplished something extraordinary.

And finally, if you've found this book useful in any way, an honest review is always appreciated!

Thank you for taking the time to read this book and good luck in your journey to a healthier you!

About the Author

ANTHEA PERIES BSC (Hons) is a published author, she completed her undergraduate studies in several branches of the sciences, including Biology, Brain and Behaviour and Child Development. A former graduate member of the British Psychological Society, she has experience in counselling and is a former senior management executive. Born in London, Anthea enjoys fine cuisine, writing, and has travelled the world.

Thank you for purchasing this book, if you found it helpful, please leave an honest review when convenient.

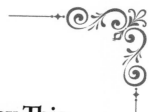

Other Books by This Author

- Food Addiction: Why You Eat to Fall Asleep and How to Overcome Night Eating Syndrome

- Food Addiction: Overcoming Your Addiction to Sugar, Junk Food, and Binge Eating

- Food Addiction: Overcome Sugar Bingeing, Overeating on Junk Food & Night Eating Syndrome

- Food Addiction: Binge Eating Disorders

- Food Addiction: Stop Binge Eating, Food Cravings and Night Eating, Overcome Your Addiction to Junk Food & Sugar

- Food Cravings: Simple Strategies to Help Deal with Craving for Sugar & Junk Food

- Overcome Food Addiction: How to Overcome Food Addiction, Binge Eating and Food Cravings

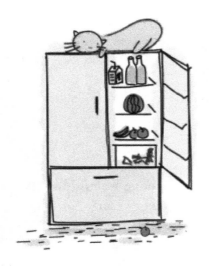

Don't miss out!

Visit the website below and you can sign up to receive emails whenever Anthea Peries publishes a new book. There's no charge and no obligation.

https://books2read.com/r/B-A-DMCG-FCLT

BOOKS 2 READ

Connecting independent readers to independent writers.

Also by Anthea Peries

Cancer and Chemotherapy

Coping with Cancer & Chemotherapy Treatment: What You Need to Know to Get Through Chemo Sessions
Coping with Cancer: How Can You Help Someone with Cancer, Dealing with Cancer Family Member, Facing Cancer Alone, Dealing with Terminal Cancer Diagnosis, Chemotherapy Treatment & Recovery
Chemotherapy Survival Guide: Coping with Cancer & Chemotherapy Treatment Side Effects

Eating Disorders

Food Cravings: Simple Strategies to Help Deal with Craving for Sugar & Junk Food
Sugar Cravings: How to Stop Sugar Addiction & Lose Weight
The Immune System, Autoimmune Diseases & Inflammatory Conditions: Improve Immunity, Eating Disorders & Eating for Health
Food Addiction: Overcome Sugar Bingeing, Overeating on Junk Food & Night Eating Syndrome

Food Addiction: Overcoming your Addiction to Sugar, Junk Food, and Binge Eating

Food Addiction: Why You Eat to Fall Asleep and How to Overcome Night Eating Syndrome

Overcome Food Addiction: How to Overcome Food Addiction, Binge Eating and Food Cravings

Healthy Gut: Transform Your Health from the Inside Out, for a Healthy You

Emotional Eating: Stop Emotional Eating & Develop Intuitive Eating Habits to Keep Your Weight Down

Emotional Eating: Overcoming Emotional Eating, Food Addiction and Binge Eating for Good

Food Addiction

Overcoming Food Addiction to Sugar, Junk Food. Stop Binge Eating and Bad Emotional Eating Habits

Food Addiction: Overcoming Emotional Eating, Binge Eating and Night Eating Syndrome

Grief, Bereavement, Death, Loss

Coping with Loss & Dealing with Grief: Surviving Bereavement, Healing & Recovery After the Death of a Loved One

How to Plan a Funeral

Health Fitness

How To Avoid Colds and Flu Everyday Tips to Prevent or Lessen The Impact of Viruses During Winter Season

Quark Cheese
50 More Ways to Use Quark Low-fat Soft Cheese: The Natural Alternative When Cooking Classic Meals
Quark Cheese Recipes: 21 Delicious Breakfast Smoothie Ideas Using Quark Cheese
30 Healthy Ways to Use Quark Low-fat Soft Cheese

Standalone
Family Style Asian Cookbook: Authentic Eurasian Recipes: Traditional Anglo-Burmese & Anglo-Indian
Coping with Loss and Dealing with Grief: The Stages of Grief and 20 Simple Ways on How to Get Through the Bad Days

About the Author

Anthea Peries BSc (Hons) is a published author, she completed her undergraduate studies in several branches of the sciences including *Biology, Neurology, Brain and Behaviour and Child Development*. A former graduate member of the *British Psychological Society*, she has experience in counselling and is a former senior management executive. Born in London, Anthea enjoys fine cuisine, writing, and has travelled the world.